THE
TOOTH DECAY
SOLUTION

How to Naturally Cure Tooth Decay and
Avoid Dental Surgery

Sandi Lane

ISBN-10: 1533243824
ISBN-13: 978-1533243829

DEDICATION

This book is dedicated to those in search of better ways of understanding teeth growth and dental liabilities or abnormalities.

CONTENTS

INTRODUCTION

Tooth decay also known as dental caries or cavities is a common disease which affects a large percentage of the world population. It is widespread and generally occurs due to poor oral habits. It is the demineralization of tooth by the acid releasing bacteria. These acids cause the tooth to decay. The decay begins on the outer surface of the tooth and progresses to deeper layers.

It is a very common condition and can occur at any age but is more common in children and young adults. It comes about when normal bacteria of the mouth combines with acids, food particles and saliva resulting in plaque, a sticky substance that sticks to the teeth.

This book contains proven steps and strategies on how to naturally cure Tooth Decay and avoid dental surgery.

CHAPTER 1 – CHEWING ASSETS: UNDERSTANDING TEETH GROWTH AND HOW THEY BECOME LIABILITIES

An asset is something that adds value to its possessor or owner. In terms of bodily functions, the teeth are chewing assets. Without teeth, just imagine how difficult it will be for a person to digest solid foods. When an asset, for some reason, malfunctions or is unable to do what it is supposed to do, it becomes a liability.

With the high costs of dental procedures (from £18.50 to £250 in England, for example), any conscientious individual would want to make sure his or her teeth do not end up being liabilities. To better appreciate the solution to the problem of tooth decay, a good place to start would be understanding teeth growth and dental liabilities or abnormalities.

Teeth Growth

A baby isn't really born all-gums. In fact, teeth are quietly growing inside a baby's jaws (yes, jaws) since birth. The baby's tiny mouth looks all gummy for 6 months until the first baby tooth (or milk tooth) shows up at the center of the baby's lower gums. Dentists call this first tooth the lower central incisor.

A toddler will have at least nine milk teeth (or deciduous teeth) on its first birthday: four upper front teeth, four lower front teeth and its first lower molar. A toddler's first upper molar appears on the 14th month. On his 18th month, a toddler will have his upper and lower pointed teeth (canines) in place, helping him munch on meat and other solid foods easier.

Ideally, by the time children are 2 ½ to 3 years old, their set of milk teeth - 20 in all - will already be complete and will normally start dropping out before they enter grade school. Pretty much on a first-in-first-out fashion, the very first tooth that falls off is the lower central incisor. Permanent or adult teeth will have replaced all baby teeth when children reach their 12th birthday.

Towards their teenage years, young people will have a full set of 28 permanent teeth. Wisdom teeth (or third molars) grow somewhere in between a person's late teens until he or she is 25, completing a set of 32 adult teeth in all. In spite of good brushing and flossing habits, human teeth normally tend to darken once a person reaches 70. Tooth loss among adults may happen at any time as a result of sickness, injury, cigarette smoking, unhealthy eating habits or poor oral hygiene.

Dental Liabilities or Abnormalities

An abnormality or anomaly is usually detected in reference to a set of standards. Any deviation from, or alteration to, the standard is categorized as an anomaly. While a dental anomaly certainly will not put a person in jail, it increases the chances for a dental surgery more than the average bucktoothed grade-schooler would.

While dental abnormalities or liabilities can be treated and prevented through proper oral hygiene and nutrition, some anomalies are genetic, that is, hereditary or inherited.

In one of its published studies, the LSUHS School of Dentistry (LSUSD) defines dental anomaly in reference to the following:

☐ Dental Pulp: Dental pulp or tooth pulp is contained in the center of a tooth. Made up of connective tissue, blood vessels and large nerves, the dental pulp is also referred to as dental nerve or tooth nerve. It helps teeth repair themselves or remineralize by forming secondary dentins when trauma occurs. The dental pulp's receptors enable teeth to send pain messages to the brain in response to temperature changes and application of pressure. It also acts as the lifeblood of teeth as it moisturizes and nourishes them.

☐ Number of teeth: Ideally, an adult should have a complete set of 32 teeth while a child has 20. There are two ways commonly used in tooth numbering: the Universal Numbering System used by general dentists and the Palmer Notation Method, which is used by most orthodontists and oral surgeons.

a. With the Universal Numbering System, numbering of adult teeth starts with the farthest tooth on the right side of the mouth, going towards the tooth on the farthest left

(1-16). The number continues from 17-32 from the tooth on the farthest bottom left of the mouth towards the tooth on the farthest bottom right. Children's teeth are numbered following the same pattern, but with a small letter "d" (for deciduous) written beside each number. A modified kiddie version eliminates the numbers and uses uppercase letters A to T instead.

b. The Palmer Notation Method, on the other hand, divides the set of teeth into four quadrants: Upper Right (UR), Upper Left (UL), Lower Left (LL) and Lower Right (LR). Numbering begins from the front center of the mouth, going towards the back. To identify the teeth on each quadrant, the numbers 1 to 8 are used for an adult's teeth while the uppercase letters A to E are used for a child's teeth.

☐ Size of teeth: Though the concept of beauty is not absolute, it is generally considered that people whose teeth are too short tend to look older while those whose teeth are too long look gawky.

Cosmetic dentist Laurence R. Rifkin, DDS, in an interview with NewBeauty.com, revealed that while a person's central incisors or front teeth should have an 82% to 85% height-to-width proportion, teeth size varies among individuals and is directly affected by gum tissue, bone loss, inflammation or previous dental work like veneers or bonding. Before creating a more aesthetically balanced look for their patients, specialists like Dr. Rifkin make a careful evaluation to see why the teeth are either too long or too short.

☐ Shape of teeth: The ideal shape of the human teeth depends on the type of teeth and their function.

a. Incisors: Used for chopping (incising), incisors are shaped like a chisel with thin edges.

b.   Canines: Helpful in tearing through meaty food, these assets are naturally pointy and sharp.

c. Premolars: Children do not have premolars. Among adults, these grinders are shaped like a diamond and normally have wide and jagged occlusal (chewing) surfaces.

d.   Molars: Like premolars, molars are designed to grind food. They are rectangular in shape and also have wide and jagged occlusal surfaces.

☐   Position of teeth: A good way to see if a person's teeth are well-positioned is the "bite." It is directly related to how one's jaws are aligned.

☐   Enamel or Dentin: The enamel protects the dentine, which in turn protects the nerves and the dental pulp. It is said to be the hardest part in the human body; but once it chips, it doesn't regenerate because it has no blood supply. Dentine, on the other hand, reproduces in response to wear and tear.

Dental Anomalies

The Consumer Guide to Dentistry lists the following dental anomalies or abnormalities along with several other oral diseases:

Malocclusion: Take a bite. When the jaws are improperly aligned due to missing, extra or crowed teeth, malocclusion or "bad bite" happens. A person's speech, manner of chewing as well as facial appearance may be affected by this hereditary anomaly. Malocclusion is usually linked to temporomandibular jaw (TMJ) disorder. It may be corrected through a combination of surgical and orthodontic procedures to relieve pain and discomfort and resume normal eating and/or speech patterns.

Dentinogenesis Imperfecta and Amelogenesis Imperfecta: Dentinogenesis imperfecta happens when the dentin in one's teeth is not enough to build strong enamel, causing the teeth's surface to flake. Amelogenesis imperfecta takes place when the teeth en-amel fails to form fully. Persons with these two anomalies experience sensitivity to pressure and temperature. Their teeth are likely to break easily.

Supernumerary Teeth: Characterized by its odd shape, a supernumerary tooth is a tooth in excess (super-) of the normal number (-numerary) of permanent teeth. It can appear in any part of a person's mouth, but usually in the upper area. One of the recognizable forms of supernumerary teeth is mesioden, which is known for its conical crown and short root maxillary. People with cleft palate are known to have supernumerary teeth.

Hypodontia or Anodontia: Either some permanent teeth are missing (hypodontia) or all of them are missing (anodontia) because the primary (baby) teeth failed to fully develop. Some dentists may advise to just let 'unripe' baby teeth stay where they are, but there are instances when they would pull it out and put a brace in place to prevent malocclusion.

CHAPTER 2 – THE FLAGGED TOOTH

Understanding teeth growth and knowing about certain dental abnormalities help paint a picture of what an ideal set of teeth would look like. However, it may well be agreed, that anyone who has teeth is likely to be flagged or be a candidate for dental surgery or, at the very least, tooth decay.

Tooth Decay and Its Symptoms

Tooth decay is caused by acid buildup in the teeth due to, not surprisingly, an unhealthy diet. Processed food and sweets in particular leave traces of bacteria in the mouth. When the teeth are not properly or regularly cleaned, a film-like covering called plaque forms around the teeth and gums. Plaque feeds on sugar and as it feeds, it breeds acid.

The following are red flags or telltale signs of tooth decay:

• Presence of yellowish patch or tartar (hardened plaque) on teeth
  • Pain when eating sweets
  • Sensitivity to hot and cold food and drinks
  • Bad breath

Oral Hygiene Habits Checklist

For expert advice on dental health, it is always best to see a dentist or an orthodontist. Here's a checklist of questions to help assess one's oral hygiene habits:
  • Am I drinking at least eight glasses of water a day?
  • Do I floss after meals?
  • Do I brush my teeth with fluoride toothpaste at least twice a day?
  • Do I rinse my mouth with a fluoride mouthwash?
  • Am I fond of eating fruits and vegetables?
  • Do I visit the dentist at least twice a year?
  • As much as I can, do I avoid eating sugary and starchy food?
  • Do I stay away from eating processed food?

CHAPTER 3 – BRUSH, FLOSS AND PULL

Although the checklist in the preceding chapter is not exhaustive, it should give a hint on the two different approaches to dental care.

Take a look at those eight questions again and this time classify each of them under two categories: Conventional or Natural.

Conventional Methods of Tooth Care

- ☐ Brush with fluoride toothpaste at least twice a day.
- ☐ Floss after meals.
- ☐ Rinse with a fluoride mouthwash.
- ☐ Visit the dentist at least twice a year.

Natural Tooth Care

- ☐ Drink at least eight glasses of water a day.
- ☐ Avoid sugary and starch foods.
- ☐ Avoid processed foods.

☐   Eat fruits and vegetables.

Notice the difference? While conventional methods address the problem of the teeth externally, natural tooth care addresses the internal workings of the digestive system. What is the point?

The point is nutrition is essential in achieving healthy teeth. Further in this book will be two adult patients whose stories are key instruments to understanding the importance between conventional and natural approaches to dental care. From those stories, one can infer how crucial nutrition is in achieving healthier teeth and avoiding costly dental procedures altogether.

CHAPTER 4 – BITE IT OFF!

Tooth decay is inevitable and there's no way for the clock to stop ticking. Is there still hope? Is there a way to possibly resurrect a dying tooth other than having a dental filling and/or going under the knife? Is there a way to prevent the death of one's teeth?

For anyone who has a high probability of tooth decay, it is not all bad news. Though dental surgery remains to be the most common option to correct dental defects, the good news is, studies show that it isn't the only way. In fact, more and more people are discovering that there is, indeed, a natural way!

Surgery is optional as long as one's "flagged" tooth, or teeth, pose no great threat to one's optimal health. Take bucktooth for instance. It's quite cute for some, actually. If, however, the likelihood of having a dental surgery is due to one's poor oral hygiene AND eating habits, welcome to this chapter!

Changing/Improving Dental Care Habits

Admit it or not, people tend to resist change. However, when routine suffers threat or acquires failure (like a decayed tooth), a person realizes the critical need to make certain changes - adjustments - to attempt correction, redemption or prevention at the soonest possible time!

Why wait before it is, so to speak, too late? Bite off and chew on these six simple yet often-ignored conventional H-A-B-I-T-S for better dental health:

1.   Hydrate. There's no better way to jumpstart dental - and overall - health by increasing fluid intake. The Mayo Clinic refutes the habit of "8 glasses of water daily" and instead recommends people to "drink eight 8-ounce glasses of fluid a day," measuring not just water but all other fluids.

Water is, of course, still the best way to replenish one's supply of fluid to the body. Heavy workout, hot weather, illness and pregnancy are good reasons to increase water intake by at least 1.5 to 2.5 cups a day. Increasing one's hydration levels in proportion to physical needs leads to improved bodily functions from the inside out.

2.   Avoid starches and sugars. Though sugar is the most common go-to food for energy, the boosting effect of sugar is only short-term. Dependence on sugar often leads to fluctuating blood sugar levels, which leads to mood swings, fatigue, fuzzy thinking and worst, diabetes. Cutting down on one's sugar intake can actually do more good than harm. Consider this: less sugar, less plaque; no plaque, no tooth decay. It comes with weight loss as a bonus, too!

3.   Brush at least twice a day. While some dental

practitioners recommend brushing one's teeth before having breakfast, waiting at least 30 minutes after eating is also advisable. This prevents the teeth enamel from being damaged - particularly after eating sugar-rich and acidic food.

4.   Take time to brush, at least for two minutes on each instance. Hurried brushing is potentially harmful to the gums. Softly massaging the gums in addition to flossing and cleaning the tongue make up for an excellent toothbrush routine. Mouthwash? Optional.

5.   See the dentist regularly, depending on individual needs. In her report "How Often Do You Need to See a Dentist?" last September 28, 2014, the BBC's Claudia Hammond revealed that the results of several systematic researches gave no conclusive basis whether to dispute or to support the idea of six monthly check-ups. Hammond submitted that socio-economic status, availability of dental equipment and nutrition can also affect the relation between one's dental health and the frequency of dental visits. Individual risk assessment, she concluded, is a good basis for how long a patient can wait before seeing the dentist again.

Diet Adjustment

While it is almost always a universally-accepted (conventional) fact that tooth decay is attributable to poor brushing habits and oral hygiene, dental health advocate and international author Ramiel Nagel pinpoints to better nutrition as the better way to address the root cause of tooth decay.

Gleaned from the works of dentist Dr. Weston A. Price and backed by his own extensive research and personal experience over a five-year period, Nagel in his book Cure

Tooth Decay™ presents guidelines on how to naturally remineralize teeth and avoid costly dental procedures. Nagel debunks many of the conventional dental health practices and emphasizes nutrition.

To illustrate the importance of nutrition for better dental health, Nagel revealed the stories of an adult male who has never brushed his teeth and an adult female who diligently took care of her teeth since she was a young girl. It is normal to presume that the man who has never brushed his teeth would have all sorts of cavities in his mouth and the woman would, of course, have immaculate teeth. It turned out the opposite was true and it had something to do with their diets!

So what's a teeth-friendly heal-teeth diet?

CHAPTER 5 – THE HEAL-TEETH MENU

What was the secret of the man who never used a toothbrush in his lifetime, but after a session of oral prophylaxis revealed a healthy set of teeth?

His dentist revealed that the guy loved to drink milk! His diet consisted for the most part of vegetables, raw fruit, buttermilk and curdled milk or clapper. On the flip side, the cavity-laden lady who loved brushing her teeth also loved eating jellies, jams, pastries and pies to her detriment. She is fond of neither milk nor vegetables.

For a heal-teeth diet, Ramiel Nagel particularly stresses the importance of including more foods that are rich in fat-soluble vitamins into one's diet for better dental health. What are those?

Fat-soluble vitamins are Vitamins A, D, E and K. They are stored in one's fatty tissues and liver and stays in the body longer than water-soluble fats. Unlike water-soluble vitamins (Vitamin C and all the B-complex vitamins), fat-soluble vitamins do not need to be replaced daily, but are essential to overall well-being. However, excessive use – as in any other vitamin – may lead to toxicity.

Vitamin A, while best known to be responsible for excellent eyesight, is necessary in the formation of healthy teeth, a strong skeletal system, soft tissue and healthy skin. Too little Vitamin A causes poor eyesight and weakens the immune system while too much of it may lead to birth defects.

Vitamin D or the "sunshine vitamin" helps the body in the absorption of calcium, which, along with phosphate, is necessary for bone formation. People with inadequate supply of Vitamin D are known to suffer from cancer, high blood pressure, osteoporosis, lupus and gum diseases. An over-supply of Vitamin D, however, can damage the kidneys and bring about kidney stones.

Vitamin E, usually associated with "anti-ageing" products, is essential for cell function and a healthy immune system. While deficiency in Vitamin E is rare, large doses of Vitamin E are reported to have curtailed the progression of ataxia (a disease affecting the central nervous system). In general, however, high levels of Vitamin E can be linked to birth defects, bleeding, including brain hemorrhage.

Vitamin K is particularly needed in blood clotting (or "koagulation" in German) and helps promote healthy bones especially among old people. People who bruise and bleed easily are more likely to be deficient in Vitamin K.

One should keep in mind that these vitamins need to collaborate with other nutrients in order to achieve sound bodily functions. The key word to remember in any diet regimen, as always, is "balanced" – neither too little nor too much.

Menu for Maintaining Healthy Teeth

In the long run, complementing conventional methods of teeth care with natural methods like oil pulling will not be enough. Going deep down into the root cause of any health anomaly must be done by making the necessary adjustments in one's daily nutrition.

Keep in mind that while over-the-counter supplements are readily available, it may not be beneficial for everybody. It is advisable to ask for dietitian referrals from a trusted friend or family member. Consult a GP or dietitian before starting on any diet program. A dietitian would be best able to assess and customize a menu or diet plan based on an individual's pre-existing health conditions and nutrition goals.

It can also be particularly helpful to grow one's food or go organic, but if buying canned or processed foods cannot be avoided, it would be wise to spend a little extra time to examine the label and take note of the nutritional value.

Here are some of the sources of fat-soluble vitamins A, D, E, and K that can be added to one's current grocery list. While extra care has been done to include only verifiable sources in the preparation of this list, it will be best to remember that in everything, balance is the key.

Vitamin A

Apple, asparagus, beef liver, beet greens, broccoli, butternut squash, cantaloupe, carrots, celery, cheese, chili pepper, cod liver oil, collards, dandelion greens, dark chocolate, dried apricots, dried basil, dried marjoram, dried plums, eggs, fish, grapefruit, iceberg lettuce, kale, mangoes, meat, mustard greens, okra, papaya, paprika, parsley, peaches, peas, poultry, pumpkin, red bell pepper, spinach, sweet potatoes, tomatoes, turkey liver, turnip greens, watermelon, whole milk, winter squash, yoghurt

Vitamin D

Almond milk, beef liver, blackstrap molasses, bluefin tuna, bok choy (Chinese cabbage), broccoli, buttermilk, catfish, cheese, chocolate shake, cocoa, cod liver oil, cow milk, daylily flower, egg yolk, gai lan (Chinese broccoli), goat's milk, halibut, herring, kale, kefir, mackerel, margarine, mushrooms, mustard greens, navy beans, okra, orange juice, oyster, pink salmon, rice milk, salmon, sardines, seaweed, sesame seed butter, shrimp, snapper, sockeye, soy milk, strawberry shake, steelhead trout, turnip greens, white beans, yellowfin tuna

Vitamin E

Agar, almonds, asparagus, avocados, bell peppers, blackberries, broccoli, carrots, caviar, cooked taro, cooked quinoa, corn oil, dandelion greens, dried apricots, dry roasted peanuts, flax seeds, green pepper, hazelnuts, hazelnut oil, jalapeno peppers, kiwi fruit, mango, olives, olive oil, oregano, parsnips, peaches, peanut butter, peanuts, pine nuts, pumpkin, rainbow trout, red pepper, shrimp, soybean oil, spinach, spirulina, squash, sunflower oil, sunflower seeds, tofu, tomato, wheat germ oil

Vitamin K

Alfalfa sprouts, artichokes, asparagus, blackberries, blueberries, brewed coffee, broccoli, Brussels sprouts, canned carrot juice, cauliflower, celery, Chinese gooseberries, collards, cowpeas, cranberry-apple juice, cream of mushroom soup, dandelion greens, dried marjoram, grapes, iceberg lettuce, kale, kelp, kiwi fruit, leeks, miso, mung beans, mustard greens, okra, onions, oregano, parsley, pickled cucumber, pie crust, plums, prunes, pumpkin, red cabbage, rhubarb, sauerkraut, soybean oil, spinach, squash, taro leaves, turnip greens, mustard greens, watercress

As a bonus for downloading this ebook, try these simple heal-teeth recipes:

Cuccina Mela's Dark choco-tofu mousse

Cuccina Mela is an interactive kitchen nestled in a quiet village in Southeast Asia. Chef Mela, its executive chef, has formulated a recipe with health buffs in mind. Using silken tofu, dark chocolate made from fresh cacao, unflavored gelatin, stevia and strawberries, this recipe is packed with Vitamin A and D.

Begin by melting 250g of bittersweet dark chocolate in boiling water over a double boiler (or any pan with a glass/pyrex/stainless steel bowl above it). As soon as the dark chocolate melts, pour it into a blender along with 200 grams of silken tofu. Let the mixture blend until it is soft and well-combined.

Prepare 1 sachet of Knox unflavored gelatin according to package instructions. Combine gelatin with the dark choco-tofu mixture. Add 3 sachets of stevia to sweeten. Pour into cups then chill for about 30 minutes or until firm. Top with sliced strawberries, smile and serve!

Food & Wine's Caramelized Broccoli

Picking up from The American Academy of Cosmetic Dentistry's e-booklet, writer Colleen Casey, in her article "6 Foods and Recipes to Eat for Bright, Healthy Teeth", shares 6 easy to prepare teeth-friendly recipes. One of the featured recipes that the tooth fairy would sweetly recommend anytime is Food & Wine's caramelized broccoli. It is caramel minus the sugar and is packed with all four fat-soluble vitamins. It takes only 15 to 18 minutes to prepare. Here's how:

Heat 2 tablespoons of extra-virgin olive oil in a skillet and add 1 ¼ pounds of broccoli. Cover until the broccoli turns into a rich, brownish color on the bottom. After about 8 minutes, add ½ cup of water. The broccoli will get tender in about 7 more minutes and the water would have evaporated by that time.

Mix in 1 tablespoon of extra-virgin oil, 3 cloves of garlic and a pinch of crushed pepper. Cook uncovered. Once the garlic turns golden brown (in about 3 minutes, tops), remove from the skillet from the heat. Transfer the contents to a plate. Sprinkle the broccoli with a dash of salt, ground black pepper and a spray of lemon juice. Serve with a smile!

AACD's Green Tea Honey Syrup

Featured in the website of ewellnessmag is one of the recipes formulated by professional mixologists and Bittercube owners Nicholas Kosevich and Ira Koplowitz. They teamed up with the American Academy of Cosmetic Dentistry to come up with several teeth-friendly cocktails, one of which is Green Tea Honey Syrup.

Here's a tweaked version of the recipe, using stevia instead of granulated sugar: Boil ¾ cups of water in a pot then soak in 2 bags of green tea for five minutes. Dissolve half a cup of stevia and a cup of honey in half a cup of the brewed tea. Stir well until dissolved. Serve hot.

Though most teas tend to stain the teeth and erode dental enamel, green tea has less tannin – the element which promotes staining. Green tea can also prevent dental cavities and gum disease as it reduces bacteria and acid in the mouth.

Sandi Lane

CHAPTER 6 – OIL-PULLING FOR DENTAL AND OVERALL HEALTH

A great way to start healing tooth decay and complement one's overall wellness before making any diet adjustments is oil pulling. It is an ancient Ayurvedic practice, which is slowly gaining popularity amongst advocates of natural healing methods.

Oil pulling is a natural therapy to rid the body – not just the mouth – of harmful bacteria. Dr. F. Karach, MD is credited for integrating the science of oil pulling into his expertise in the field of medicine in 1992.

CNN's Sara Cheshire in her special report "Does oil pulling work?" last August 6, 2014, cautions that due to insufficient studies supporting the efficacy of oil pulling, the American Dental Association does not consider oil pulling as a replacement to brushing the teeth and flossing. Based on her interview with Dr. Amala Guha, founding president of The International Society for Ayurveda and Health, Cheshire stated that there are negative side effects when oil pulling is not done using the correct technique.

In spite of mixed results and feedback, oil pulling is gradually gaining popularity among natural health advocates and fitness buffs. Passionate wife, mom and writer Trina Holden in her personal blog shares her and her husband's awesome experience with teeth regeneration simply by swishing coconut oil. At the time she wrote her article on how to naturally heal cavities and strengthen one's teeth, she also hasn't been using toothpaste for more than a year!

Oil pulling is best done in an empty stomach and studies show that it is beneficial not only for oral health, but for one's overall wellness. It may be done thrice in a day for maximum detoxifying effects. Though generally safe and effective for people of all ages, oil pulling is not advisable for younger children who may end up swallowing the swished oil.

Oil pulling can be done initially (or radically!) by tossing away the bottle of mouthwash and replacing it with a bottle of any of these oils:

- Virgin coconut oil
- Olive oil
- Sesame oil
- Sunflower oil
- Butter oil

Of the above, coconut oil has been found by the Athlone Institute of Technology to be most beneficial for dental health as it was the only oil which, upon treatment with enzymes, successfully eliminated the bacteria Streptococcus mutans from the mouth. This bacterium is known to be a major contributor to tooth decay.

Four don'ts to remember while oil pulling:
- Don't rush. Enjoy swishing the oil in the mouth for a minimum of 3 minutes and maximum of 5 minutes, twice daily.
- Don't gargle.
- Don't swallow.
- Don't spit the oil into the sink. The oil tends to harden and clog up the drain. Spit into the toilet bowl instead.

When to oil pull:
- In the morning, before eating or drinking anything.
- 4 hours after eating.
- 1 hour after drinking.

What to prepare:
- Virgin coconut oil (or any of the recommended oils mentioned earlier), 2 tablespoons
- Water with salt, 1 glass
- Lukewarm water, 1 to 2 glasses

How to do it:
In her interview with Dr. Gaha, Sara Cheshire found out that there are actually two techniques for oil pulling: gandusa and kavala.

Gandusa: Fill the mouth with oil. Hold the oil still in the mouth for 3 to 5 minutes. Spit. Repeat for 2 to 3 times.

Kavala: Fill the mouth with oil. Hold still for 2 minutes. Swish. Spit. Repeat for 2 to 3 times.

Both techniques should last for a maximum of 5 minutes in each session.

Most of the people who share their oil pulling experiences online are actually using the kavala technique where the oil is swirled or swished around the mouth.

They do it for 10 to 20 minutes at one go.

Regardless of technique, the oil acts like a magnet, "pulling" all the harmful bacteria into it while the oil is in the mouth. This is why oil pulling is not recommended for kids who are not yet used to spitting out. Think of all the bacteria that they will end up swallowing instead of expelling!

After spitting out the oil, rinse the mouth with salt-infused water and spit. Drink lukewarm water afterwards.

What to expect:

When improperly done, according to Dr. Gaha, oil pulling may have negative side effects including temporary loss of taste or sensation in the mouth, dry mouth, muscular stiffness and excessive thirst.

Dr. Bruce Fife, author of "Oil Pulling for a Brighter Smile and Better Health", advises that mucus might build up at the back of the throat while swishing. When this happens, the oil should be expelled first. Then the mucus should be coughed out of the throat. Resume oil pulling by taking another tablespoon of oil and swish until the process is completed.

The cure may not be readily evident and the symptoms may, in fact, get worse during the first few days while on oil pulling therapy. It shouldn't be a cause for alarm because it is a part of the detoxification or healing process.

With regular use, aside from its many benefits to one's overall health and wellness, oil pulling is known to heal dental cavities, remove plaque, reduce swollen gums, strengthen the jaws, whiten the teeth and eliminate bad breath.

Please Leave a Review

Finally, if you enjoyed this book, please take the time to share your thoughts and post a review. It would be greatly appreciated.

That review and feedback will help me improve the content in my books – and make each and every one more relevant and helpful to you.

Thank you again and good luck!

Sandi Lane